CREATING

IN DANGEROUS TIMES

CELESTE NAZELI SNOWBER

Creating in Dangerous Times

Celeste Nazeli Snowber
Copyright ©2025

Published in Canada by HARP The People's Press
216 Clydesdale Road, Clydesdale, Nova Scotia B2G 2K9
www.tryhealingarts.ca

Canadian Cataloguing in Publication Data
ISBN 978-1-990137-73-0

Cover Art: Barbara Houston
Cover Design: Micah Schroeder
Book Layout: Greg Walsh

The Circle of Abundance Indigenous Program, Coady International Institute, St. Francis Xavier University: www.coady.stfx.ca/circle-of-abundance; and David Suzuki Foundation (one nature): www.davidsuzuki.org receive 20% of sales, distributed equally

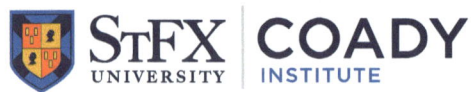 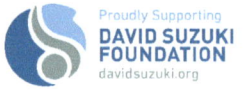 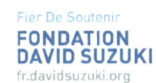

In Praise of *Creating in Dangerous Times*

Creating in Dangerous Times is evocative, timely and timeless, a celebration of creativity. Author Celeste Snowber remains a master of inspiration, motivation and challenge. Every word, prose and verse, is poetic and sensory, the depth of engagement one associates with a flawless culinary experience, one we only wish could last longer.

> — **Bill Arnott**, bestselling author of *A Perfect Day for a Walk* and the *Season* memoirs.

Celeste Snowber has written a heart opening book, with poems of beauty to help us through. Calling forth a remembering to live and create, fully, vividly, with an eagerness to embrace the fullness of our lives. Delicious, inspired and inspiring!

> — **Margie Gillis**, OC solo dancer and choreographer, Margie Gillis Dance Foundation

In *Creating in Dangerous Times,* Celeste speaks to the depths of all that I can/not access inside myself. She shakes loose what I have so tightly contained and holds with care all that I am afraid to release. This text is a collection of remedies to living in a world that has forgotten the richness of life. It is a gift, a provocation, a plea, and a prayer. Re/imagine yourself through her words and re/discover the alchemy within your humanness.

> — **Ellyn Lyle**, Dean and Professor, Cape Breton University

At a time when we need them most, Celeste Snowber's wise and gentle words offer both solace and strength. These provocations, borne of empathy and connection, are brimming with hope and humanity.

> — **Lorri Neilsen Glenn**, author of *The Old Moon in Her Arms: Women I Have Known and Been.*

Creating in Dangerous Times is a powerful invitation to embrace artistry, embodiment, and resilience. With deep wisdom and poetic grace, Celeste Snowber reminds us that even amidst uncertainty, we can create, move, and live fully. In a world longing for connection and authenticity, her work offers a vital path to creativity and presence.

> — **Jodi Proznick**, award winning bassist, composer, educator, producer

In a world drunk on productivity and gripped in the tyranny of the urgent, this book is a provocation and invitation to s l o w down. Take these templates, infuse them with your starved senses, your thirsty images, your urgent dreams, until you carve a temple of presence and renewal, until you allow the possible to dance with the impossible. Repeat daily.

> — **Daniela Elza**, author of *SCAR/CITY* and *Is This an Illness or an Accident?* (2025)

Also by Celeste Nazeli Snowber

Dance, place and poetics: Site-specific performance as a portal to knowing

The marrow of longing

Blue waiting (co-authored)

Embodied inquiry: Writing, living and being through the body

Wild tourist: Instructions to a wild tourist from the divine feminine

Landscapes in aesthetic education (co-authored)

In the womb of God: Creative nurturing for the soul

Embodied prayer: Towards wholeness of body, mind, soul

Contents

INVITATION

Creativity is our birthright as human beings. We need
to remember and rebody what we were made for.
In these uncertain times, we need to invoke courage
and preserve our inner wildness and return to the
wilderness of our souls. We need to reclaim our
birthright and migrate back to the life that is calling
to us.

We live in dangerous times. There is a crisis of the
imagination. This takes shape in a myriad of ways.
We have forgotten how to access our whole beings
as central to the act of creating. We need to live
artfully to sustain the whole planet, and to sustain
ourselves—these are connected. We cannot open
generative spaces unless we access our own wellness.
As we draw from the inspiration that is rooted in
what it means to be truly human, we cultivate the
connections between body, soul, mind and heart.
Here lies our hope.

Inspiration is closer to us than we know. Present
when we inhale and exhale. How do we stay
inspired when all that we breathe in is the tyranny
of the urgent? What if we responded to the call
to both honour and embrace all of who we are in
our humanness? A broken heart is a place to begin
again. Fragility is the terroir for transformation.
Vulnerability is a superpower. Being human is
drawing on the humus, humour and humility intrinsic
to our whole selves. Remember, we are paradoxical
and wonderous beings.

What if we could show up for all the parts of our lives—grief or elation, disappointment or satisfaction, and bring the wisdom of our bodies to our journey of living creatively? The body is the portal to creativity. To live through the senses, whether it is an intuitive knowing in the gut, or being wide-awake, is to nurture creativity. There is a dance inviting you to reconnect creativity, physicality and spirituality. The physical world is shot through with the pulse of the holy. You too, are beckoned to the pulse of your own voice being expressed.

Creating in Dangerous Times is designed for all creatives—artists and scientists, dancers and doctors, musicians and scholars, inventors and influencers, dreamers, seekers and mystics. This book comes out of my own life, finding ways to live creatively in the midst of many demands and challenges. We all have them, and that's what it means to be human. Life is faithful to bring suffering. *Creating in Dangerous Times* is an offering. A companion to help unfold what has always been within you.

I invite you, as a reader, to ponder the questions rising within you.

Dare to make an appointment with your creativity.

PROVOCATION

Doubt and the imposter syndrome will follow you.
I always say that when I get resistance, and this
happens often, I know I am on the right track.
Nothing I have ever wanted to accomplish has come
without difficulty and wonder. In writing this book,
I let my questions become a place for alchemy. I am
given boldness to show up for my own life. In turn,
I offer these poetic meditations and invite you to be
compassionate towards all that arises within you, even
your own resistance.

You can read them in any order; sit with just a few
of them with morning coffee or tea. See them as a
mini retreat to reboot your creative life. We all need
reminders to rebody our deepest yearning. They are
given to nourish your creativity.

Over the years I have integrated these meditations
in my own teaching and mentoring practices. Many
times, we can get stuck in our writing. Let these
poetic prompts be a springboard to release what is
within you. Discover the unknown. Integrate them in
your own practices in community, so others too can
be inspired by what is calling to them.

Let these be provocations to live more deeply into the
life that wants to be lived in you. Think of them as
Matins for creating, a bell to call you to attend to your
inner birdsong. May you bear witness to your own
becoming. Even in dangerous times.

welcome

welcome all the parts of yourself
to the page, to the studio, to the home
inside

so the branches of your fragility
synapses of your neurons
exaltations and wounds
can give voice to creation

befriend the stranger within
who is pleading for an audience
wants to come out and play
with all of who you are

no matter the size of the talent
greatness of skill
availability of time
each small creative act
is an act of courage

leap into the unknown
where what is inside
meets the world
shattered, fragile, broken
   precious, luminous

in all things
we exist, we create

we re-create

what if you stepped
into your own life
and began to love
all the pages
you

      t

        u

          r

            n

              e

                d

in your
own personal story?

living

living creatively
living artistically
living poetically
living musically

is also part of making art

the listening and living
attending fully
is the curriculum

for nourishing the creative

risk

allow the possible
to dance with the impossible

all in a spiraling

      from one part
      of the self to the other

where risk lives

wholeness resides

list

- notice the sky
- watch the fuchsia on the patio and wait till the hummingbird comes
- rotate your feet in circles, release your neck
- saunter till you find birdsong or it finds you
- write a list of ideas to dream
- write one-sentence stories of each dream
- lie on the ground outside
- let the earth support you
- begin your dreams

breath

could there be
a climate change
to creativity?

pay attention
to what restores
so inner space for the creative

can b r e a t h e

an inhale,
an exhale

the breath of what may arise

witness

bear witness
to your own becoming

give into the life
that wants to
be lived
in you

slowdance

take your pen and paintbrush
hands, feet, voice and belly
let them slowdance with you

      form the visible
      from the invisible

art making is

the great love story

travel to your inner sanctum
where there is a blank space

for what may emerge

walk, swim, dance, paddle
even twiddle your thumbs

whatever delights you

      sanctums can be places
of stillness and movement

what lies there
      is the delicious sacred

of you and the divine
however you articulate

creating awaits

unfurl

sometimes the creative path
is getting up and brushing your teeth
hydrating your body
then attending to a few small things

a dance of 60 seconds
writing for 5 minutes
pondering the sky

if you do this for a year
you'll have a performance
a book, and deep affection
for the sky

migrate

migrate to your own creativity
waiting patiently for you
to come home
and be held
in its arms

fragility

fragile derives from *frangere*
meaning *to break*

when we break open, split
new colors can be born

pliable, flexible, porous
pieces are scattered

one of those fragments
can hold
a world

make room for fragility

dare

write
 what you dare not write
dance
 what you dare not dance
create
 what you dare not create

places hidden
 in your bones
where longing resides

your dreams ache
 to arrive
be massaged

to birth

unseen

as molecules cannot be seen
with the naked eye
the unseen guides you
more than you know

here is a force
working beneath the layers
of the visible

something that can only
be imagined
lies in the door/way
until it is ready to come forth

respirate

inhale and exhale
create and recreate

    where blood turns to ink
    breath to movement
    sweat to syllables

breathe through listening
        to responding

transport the sublime

alter

cooperate with your own nature

are you a willow
        or a western red cedar
are you a mountain stream
        or rugged coastal waters

accept and celebrate your own texture
this is the only thing you can
        do anything about

you can't always alter circumstances
but you can alter your relation to them

place them on the altar

        and they will be altered

w o m b

there are days one wants to retreat
into a womb   womb days

remember   this is where you were
created

to be creative again
you must retreat there

let your fragility be held
brittleness softened
tiredness restored

drink the food of quiet
where only the wind is heard
and spirit is felt

silence

live out loud

from a deep place

of silence

midwife

it is easy to attend
        to mentoring others

but there is a time
        to mentor yourself

no one else can do the work
        you are called to

do not miss who you will become

midwife your own
life and art

porous

stay open
let part of you

      b r e a t h e into what may arrive

expect epiphanies
to birth in your flesh

where a new pathway
      hydrates

what is longing for a return

to know you were made to create
      to live
      to feel deeply

nurture perforations

stay porous

practice

i'm a bold woman living out loud
but it's the subtle actions that cause change
day after day

pen to page
torso to movement, hand to strings
daily   weekly

you must feed your body daily
daily feed your soul –
the soul who longs
to create, play, exist
into a fresh pause
when walking into wonder
is a practice

creating reminds us
where to turn

listen to desire
let impulse have its way

stop
what you are doing
      writing an email, planning an event,
      scrolling your phone

take pause, get up

turn
      spin
            move

to one new word, idea, gesture
that calls for
attention

listen

listen to the cadence
of your body

hear

the hymn of your own heart

listen to your own

birdsong

spill

drink

from your own deep well

and   s
          p
            i
             l
              l

              when necessary

solitude

reside in the call
to your true self
alone, but full
of a world running
through your senses

let silence nourish
what is within

your dreams and emotions

the score of your life
needs to be heard

solitude is the overture
for new beginnings

luxuriate

your senses are a feast
alone or together
they may lead you
in the knowing you need

trust your body
luxuriate in smells
touch the earth
and listen for buds
to push through

you are fertile soil

softness

let the softness of fog
blanket you
        calling you to a rest
that is seeking you out

here is a womb
        to retreat in

how can we start listening
        to our song again

stopping to hold the nuances
waiting to arrive

tenderness is the train
        that is coming for you

get a ticket to organic replenishment
        your body seeks

could rest be as important
      as productivity

could rest be the soil
      for seeds to grow

germinating ideas

      so they replenish

trust the landscape of tiredness

      inviting you to sabbath

abide in not doing

fast

what if we took a fast
from striving, believed
          in another way

where awe is at the centre
the notes of a new music

soaked in the silence
of becoming

face it: we are all overloaded
over the load

go under the covers, the light,
          the pillows, the shadows

take yourself for tea
          in the middle of the afternoon
and leave your technology home
put it to bed

and wait

there is much more to fast from

fast into a pause

halt

make more time
     to halt
     to live poetically

slow down and enter
dream space

     be the art
     you crave

solace

cherish solace
        the lace sewn
in your memory

thread stillness
        into the fabric
of your becoming

not producing
can be productive

let rest guide you

u n / s t u c k

be compassionate
            towards your stuckness

this too is necessary
a resting place for your thoughts

to sit on their own mat

don't bully your budding creation
            however it may take shape

it too is a child of unknowing

the s
        l
          a
            n
              t

of the creator

hidden in the elbow of

your dancing legs,
        writing arms,
                spinning mind

gentleness and fierceness
are companions

foster each in this tango

here you will be

stuck and unstuck

appointment

you make an appointment
with the dentist, doctor, accountant
make an appointment
with your muse

give her, him, them a slot for speaking

otherwise

no appointments

become disappointments

choose

you don't choose
a creative path

    it chooses you

and then

    you must choose it
    over and over again

    and say

y e s

making

an artwork is a meal
one offers to the world

if no one sits at the table
was it still worth making?

who are we to judge
what can happen

    to a creation
    a book, painting, dance, poem

just keep making

offer

persistence

there is
a connection

to creativity
      that never lets go
      of us

a lover
      who is quiet
      and
      also roars

align

we wait for the stars to align
sometimes we are away
from our star: *desiderare*
to desire comes from

    "await what the stars will bring"

so

we do our work
scribble, sing, soar
compose, cry, choreograph
weave, wait, weld

and the stars align

compost

return to what is within
waiting to be loved into
the next chapter

love unfinished projects
with tenderness; nurture
them to existence

or let them sit
even bury them
honouring their potential

compost
for what is to come

vulnerability is
       your superpower

let the salt of tears
       become prayers
let decay become
       seeds for beauty

a conduit to be brave

       to be authentic
       is an artwork

this too is a toolkit

for expression

r (eject) i o n

if you are an artist, writer, performer
and put your work out
it will be rejected
and one point or another

multiples losses

eject yourself
from the rejection

audition, place, send your work
somewhere else

this is part of the game
keep creating

land somewhere else

falling

practice falling
a necessary movement
dancers know this
to release, to rise
one must fall

it is the place in-between
where we live
each gesture is holy
an ever-changing
falling and rising

hormones and inspiration
have more in common
than we may admit

both are always present
in the body

and both

      have their own mind

creating is not polite
clothed in formal wear
dressed for a ball or prom

but comes on wild horses
on the edge of waves
disruptive as a storm
luscious as green moss

and then in the stillness
of a clear lake

creativity is honed, edited
formed and transformed
to what it asks
to become

creativity insists

wild

to access
    the wild

one must access

the shadows

constellations

you can hear the stars speak
you know there are constellations

      within you   an expanse of solitude

sometimes it feels like an agitation

      to experience more
      than what you know
      or where you can go
      a restlessness with your own star home

you are made up
of earth and sky
mud and sapphire mingled
in the heart of you

what would it mean to praise
    paradox?

paradoxology is what you find

    where duality lives

either/or/both/and
    are

    ingredients for a life

here is another wisdom

    call it what you want
    but its within and beyond

this is not a linear path

paradoxology: to praise paradox

howl

sometimes all we can do is howl

empty the lungs, breathe deep
every distraction is another
attraction to listen

to what is within
your unconscious, imperceptible
at times, and then as close
as your lover's breath

let all run through you
whispers and howls

awaken your voice

faith

there will always be demands, deadlines,
        heartaches, bills

the tyranny of the urgent

your one precious life
waits for you
as a faithful lover

it takes faith
        to leap into an empty page
        canvas, studio, kitchen

what is within you
becomes greater when
you offer it a material home

faith is a muscle

limits

you can grow vegetables
weeds, pounds, inches or poems
but how does one grow grace?

restrictions and limits are recipes
to work with what seems impossible
and then a tiny
opening
becomes a portal

one walks, sways, dances
through and beyond,
until mystery sits at your feet
rises through the body
and becomes the possible

interruptions

if you chart something
it runs the risk
of being cancelled, interrupted,
postponed or disrupted

but one can't diminish
the power of creativity

always

burning, smoldering
in the embers

sometimes the interruption
is exactly the fire
to ignite
the next song, poem, plan,
idea or dance

waiting to erupt

pressure

there are many kinds of pressure:

      internal and external
      financial and emotional
      familial and social

let yourself be drawn
to what inspires

it may not always be the recipe
      to success or reason

creativity has its own reasons
      fermenting in the soul
      wanting to rise

pressing to surety
in the clamour

listen to your own resistance
it is a teacher
where your existence is
      calling, beckoning

become dancing partners
with your own resistance

and let it lead you to
      resist(d)ance

know
      when resistance

comes your way

you are on track

more

you plan to create one project
set aside time, gather notes, research
sketch, doodle, dream, dabble

but all you can think of is another
            idea, form, blooming inside

you may feel you are betraying
your original love
polyamorous creativity   multiple births
sometimes occur

make room for what
you thought was impossible

dream more

how does one grow courage

> when defeat, disappointment, hardship
> wear down the bones of the heart?

> *courage* comes from the word *heart*

do seagulls ask themselves
> "dare we fly today?"

they cooperate with their own nature

what are the obstacles to courage?

what if we wrote, danced, dreamed, dared

knowing our lives depended on it?

disrupt
your expectations

of even what each creative idea
        may form or become

give permission for disruption
        interruption and rupture

they might be the

crack that breaks open
        a light than cannot
be extinguished

paddle

you may be paddling alone
        but you are paddling with angels

there are many in your life
holding you in an embrace

        recognize the community

        of saints in your midst

even the ones

who annoy you

what grounds us
can be portals to loss
grief of loved ones
disappointments, multiplied

a rose in winter

what defies purpose
is sometimes random

an opening
is a closure
a closure
is an opening

danger is an opportunity

fallow

there is a season for slowing
down to the roots of dormancy
let winter have its way
through the fibres of fingers
which give themselves to create

t r u s t fallow time

expect less
observe
ruminate as a task

prepare

        your whole body
        for a blank slate

a still opening

detours

there are as many detours
as trails for your feet

some may change you
forever

presenting a pathway

        to the life
        that yearns to be lived
        through you

a portal for the holy

formed

in the mundane

pregnant

there is a world
inside your body
waiting to be borne

your task:

feed what moves
          in your
womb, hips, pelvis

till your throat sings
fingers write, toes dance

more importantly

honour each pain
this too is part of creation

awaiting a new birth

time

you
need time

for the petals inside
your body

> d
> l
>   o
>   f
>   n
> u
> to

steep

what you steep yourself in

      is who you will become

if you steep yourself in beauty

you will become

beauty

known

creativity
wants to be known

through us

gratitude

a long fatigue
is this aging?

or just not living in the rhythm
you are being called to?

eat the alphabet of gratitude
here are the syllables

which provide
an antidote

danger

at the heart of danger
        is paradox

danger is a terrible
        disrupter

one cannot stay still
        it is a call to turn

pivot to your heart's purpose

before you

is the next step

excess

sometimes more is
        not more

less can be more

to access more
        let go of the excess

hundreds of pages
        yield ten meaningful ones

a whole harvest of tomatoes
may only have a few juicy ones

some creations are for your eyes only

others will meet the world
and go on their journey

be faithful to the life
    that wants to be lived
    through you
    only by you

the stories you have lived
are the material for
    making
    unmaking
    remaking

the creativity
    to flow through your body
    to others

be faithful to
    your own story

garden

your art is a garden
your life is a garden

each day we need watering

     replenish the source

making is the practice

return

keep creating

in dangerous times

keep announcing
the naked bold beauty
to the world
even in the heartbreak
horrors and injustices

so we can all
remember
what we are destined for

to live as creatures of love
awake to each moment

as the gift it was
given

ACKNOWLEDGMENTS

I acknowledge that I am a visitor on this earth, and in particular, I create, play, work, dance and write on the unceded, traditional and ancestral lands of the Halkomelem speaking peoples.

I'm grateful to Dorothy Lander and John Graham-Pole who had the initial vision to start HARP Publishing and connect the arts to healing. It is an absolute joy to work with them and I'm filled with appreciation. Thank you to Robin Grant at HARP who is a pleasure to work with.

I am in gratitude to all those people who took the time to read and respond with such beautiful and amazing endorsements. I am forever grateful for all of you, who birth creativity in fertile ways through everything you do— Bill Arnott, Daniela Elza, Margie Gillis, Lorri Neilsen Glenn, Ellyn Lyle, and Jodi Proznick. I am deeply honoured that your words accompany this book which is my heartsong.

Thank you to artist Barbara Houston for her beautiful painting on the cover.

Thank you to my son Micah Schroeder for his wonderful design of the cover.

Thank you to *Red Fern Review* for publishing some excerpts that now appear in *Creating in Dangerous Times*.

A big shout out to my dear friend and esteemed poet Susan McCaslin for our long creative friendship and for reading an initial draft.

Thanks to the audiences over the years who have been supportive as these poems were spoken and danced in various venues. Gratitude to my students who have responded to these poems as a prompt for their own writing.

Honouring my parents, Grace and Frank Snowber, who lived passionately in everything they did; infusing creativity in my veins from an early age. In turn, my heart is enlarged by my three sons, Lucas, Micah and Caleb Schroeder who keep creating in challenging times.

A special thanks with all of my being, to my beloved husband Shawn C. Brouwer who had his eye on the final drafts of this book and gave me perceptive and insightful feedback. Each day is precious living with you, where the only rule is love.

ABOUT THE AUTHOR

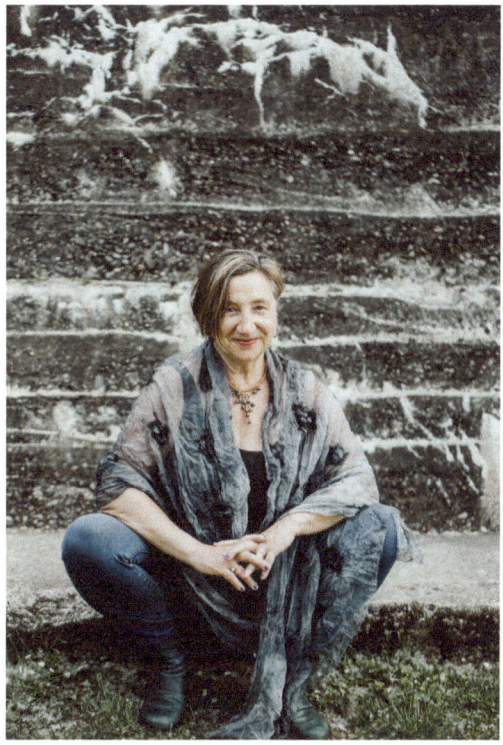

Photo credit: Michele Mateus

Celeste Nazeli Snowber, PhD is a dancer, poet, writer and award-winning educator who is a Professor in the Faculty of Education at Simon Fraser University. She has published and performed widely and her many books include: *Embodied Inquiry: Writing, living and being through the body; Dance, Place and Poetics: Site-specific performance as a portal to knowing;* and three collections of poetry. Her book of poetry, *The Marrow of Longing,* also published by HARP, explores her Armenian identity. She has performed and spoken internationally in concert venues, galleries, museums, conferences, and in various outdoor spaces. Celeste can be found at www.celestesnowber.com or more ideally, dancing between land and sea.